The Super foods Diet for Weight loss

Based on super and zero calories foods

By Glen Goodrum

Disclaimer

You Need to Tailor Your Diet to Yourself

Using your goal weight, the weight you want to be, figure out how much protein you daily needUsing your goal weight, the weight you want to be, figure out how much good oils you need.

Using your goal weight, the weight you want to be, figure out how much good carbohydrates per day you need.

Those three put together will be your daily dieting goal using the super and zero calories foods, simple, not really. But you can do it, get family members to help or friends, maybe your doctor or dietitian would help. It doesn't hurt to ask.

You are more likely to stay on and lose weight on a diet that you have put together for yourself.

Ask each family member to do the same for themselves so they know how much they should be eating.

Don't try to force them to diet, but by helping you, at least they will know when they are overeating. Plus they will have the knowledge to start if do ever start dieting. If they are agreeable they could use the Golden Diet based on 80 super foods.

When I hit a plateau where I stop losing weight, I switch over to the Golden Diet based on 80 super foods. When my body tells me to I go back on the weight loss diet. It's more important to me to remain healthy than quick weight loss.

If you eat meat try to use organic range feed meats. If you can't go on the three days water fast once a year. If your a vegetarian go organic. If you can't go on the three days water fast once a year don't worry about it.

Most people need around 1 gram of protein per kg of body weight per day. To calculate your requirements, you first need to find your weight in kg. Take your weight in weight in lbs and divide by 2.2. Now you, have your weight in kg, which is the same number of grams of protein most of us need per day.

Using that formula, a 140 lb woman would require about 64 grams of protein and a 170 lb man would require about 77 grams of protein per day."

 Researchers say too much protein can cause nausea, cramps, headaches, fatigue and bloating. That is why it's important to know how much protein you need daily and set it as the starting point for your diet. Everything else can be vegetables and fruits.

Dehydration is also a risk when you eat too much protein. If you increase your protein, you also have to increase your fluid intake. For the average person 60 to 70 ounces of water a day, which translates into eight 8-ounce glasses of water or liquid per day?

Energy: Fat is an excellent energy source. It provides 9 calories per gram, whereas protein and carbohydrates each provide 4 calories per gram.

Between 20% and 35% of your calories should come from fat.

Carbohydrates provide 45 to 65 percent of your daily calorie intake.

So if you eat a 2000-calorie diet, you should aim for about 225 to 325 grams of carbohydrates per day.

But if you need to lose weight, you will get much faster results eating around 50 to 150 grams of carbohydrates.

Foods for losing weight. Foods That Contain Almost Zero Calories that provide the energy that your body needs to function and stay alive.

If you're trying to decrease your total calorie intake, eating more low-calorie foods, such as certain fruits and vegetables, is an easy way to achieve that goal.

Here are foods with almost zero calories.

Apples

Apples are highly nutritious. One cup of apple slices has 57 calories and almost three grams of fiber. I now eat apples every day in all types of ways, its fun trying to come up with new nutritious ways to use raw apples.

Arugula

Arugula is a dark, leaf green with a pepper flavor.

It's used in salads, rich in vitamin K and also has folate, calcium and potassium. One-half cup has only three calories.

Asparagus

Asparagus is a vegetable that comes in green, white and purple colors. All types of asparagus are good for you.

One cup has 27 calories and is rich in vitamin K and foliate.

Beets

Beets are a root vegetable that have a deep-red or purple color. One of the benefits of beets is lower blood pressure.

Beets contain 59 calories per cup and potassium.

Broccoli

Broccoli is one of the most nutritious vegetables and may help fight cancer. One cup of broccoli has 31 calories and 100% of the vitamin C needs each day.

Broth

There are a number of broths, chicken, beef and vegetable. It can be eaten by itself or used as a base for soups and stews. One cup 7 to 12 calories.

Brussels sprouts

Brussels sprouts are very nutritious vegetables. They look like small cabbages and can be eaten raw or cooked.

Research shows that Brussels sprouts are high vitamin C.

They have 38 calories per cup.

Cabbage

Cabbage has green or purple leaves. It's used in slaws and salads. Is also known as sauerkraut a fermented cabbage.

It's very low in calories and has only 22 calories per cup.

Carrots

Carrots are very popular vegetables. High in vitamin A.

A cup of carrots has only 53 calories.

Cauliflower has become popular as a substitute for higher- carbohydrates vegetables and grains.

One cup of cauliflower has 25 calories and only five grams of carbohydrates.

Celery

Celery is one of the most well-known, low-calorie foods.

Its long, green stalks contain insoluble fiber that may go undigested through your body, thus contributing no calories.

Celery also has a high water content, making it naturally low in calories. There are only 18 calories in one cup of chopped celery.

Chard

Chard is a leafy green that comes in several varieties. It's extremely high in vitamin K, a nutrient that helps with proper blood clotting. One cup of chard has only 7 calories and contains 374% of vitamin K.

Clementines

Clementines resemble mini oranges. They're a common snack in the United States and are known for their high vitamin C content. One fruit packs 60% of the DV for vitamin C and only 35 calories.

Cucumbers

Cucumbers are a refreshing vegetable commonly found in salads. They're also used to flavor water along with fruits and herbs. Since cucumbers are mostly water, they're very low in calories — one-half cup only has 8.

Fennel

Fennel is a bulbous vegetable with a faint licorice taste. Dried fennel seeds are used to add an anise flavor to dishes.

Fennel can be enjoyed raw, roasted or braised. There are 27 calories in one cup of raw fennel.

Garlic

Garlic has a strong smell and taste and is used widely in cooking to add flavor to dishes. Garlic has been used for centuries as a remedy for various illnesses. Research suggests that it may decrease blood pressure and fight infections or even cancer. One clove of garlic has only 5 calories.

Grapefruit

Grapefruits are one of the most delicious and nutritious citrus fruits. They can be enjoyed on their own or on top of yogurt, salad or even fish. Certain compounds in grapefruit may decrease cholesterol levels and increase metabolism.

There are 52 calories in half a grapefruit.

Iceberg Lettuce

Iceberg lettuce is known for its high water content. It's commonly used in salads and on top of burgers or sandwiches. Even though most people think it's not as nutritious as other lettuces, iceberg lettuces is rich in vitamin K, vitamin A and foliate. One cup of iceberg lettuce has only 10 calories.

Jicama

Jicama is a tuber vegetable that resembles a white potato. This vegetable is typically eaten raw and has a texture similar to a crisp apple. One cup of jicama has over 40% of vitamin C and 46 calories.

Kale

Kale is a leafy green that has gained popularity in recent years for its impressive nutritional benefits. You can find kale in salads, smoothies and vegetable dishes.

Kale is one of the richest sources of vitamin K in the world. One cup has only 34 calories.

Lemons and Limes

The juice of lemons and limes are widely used to flavor water, salad dressings, marinades and alcoholic drinks.

Lemon juice has compounds that act as antioxidants to fight and prevent diseases. One fluid ounce of lemon or lime juice has only 8 calories.

White Mushrooms

Mushrooms are a type of fungus with a sponge-like texture. Vegetarians and vegans sometimes use them as a substitute for meat. Mushrooms contain several important nutrients and have only 15 calories per cup.

Onions are a popular vegetable.

Varieties of onions include red, white and yellow, as well as spring onions. Even though the taste differs depending on the type, all onions have very few calories one medium onion has around 44 calories.

Peppers

Peppers come in many colors, shapes and sizes. Popular types include bell peppers and jalapeños peppers. Bells peppers are high in antioxidants. Only 46 calories in one cup.

Papaya

Papaya is an orange fruit with black seeds that resembles a melon and is typically grown in tropical regions. It's very high in vitamin A and a good source of potassium. One cup of papaya has only 55 calories.

Radishes

Radishes are crunchy root vegetables with a somewhat spicy bite. They're typically seen in grocery stores as dark-pink or red but can be grown in a variety of colors. Radishes have a number of beneficial nutrients and only 19 calories per cup.

Romaine Lettuce

Romaine lettuce is a very popular leafy vegetable used in salads and on sandwiches. The calorie content of romaine is very low since it's high in water and rich in fiber. One leaf of romaine lettuce has just a one calorie.

Rutabaga

Rutabaga is a root vegetable. It tastes similar to turnips and is a good substitute for potatoes in recipes to lower the number of carbohydrates. One cup of rutabaga has 50 calories and only 11 grams of carbohydrates.

Strawberries

Strawberries are one of the most popular fruits. They're used in breakfast dishes, baked goods and salads. Berries help protect you from chronic diseases. One cup of strawberries is about 50 calories

Spinach

Spinach is leafy green that is packed with vitamins and minerals and low in calories. It is high in vitamin K, vitamin A and foliate. One-cup of spinach has only 7 calories.

Sugar Snap Peas

Sugar snap peas are a delicious variety of peas. Their pods are entirely edible and have a sweet flavor. They're typically eaten raw on their own or with a dip, yet can also be added to vegetable dishes and salads. Snap peas are highly nutritious and contain almost 100% of vitamin C. Only 41 calories in one cup.

Tomatoes

Tomatoes are one of the world's most popular vegetables. They can be eaten raw, cooked or pureed into a tomato sauce. They are highly nutritious and contain a compound called lycopene. Research has shown that lycopene may protect against cancer, inflammation and heart disease. One cup of cherry tomatoes has only 27 calories.

Turnips

Turnips are white root vegetables with a slightly bitter taste. They're often added to soups and stews. Turnips have several beneficial nutrients and only 37 calories per cup.

34. Watercress

Watercress is a leafy vegetable that grows in running water. It's typically used in salads and sandwiches. Even though watercress is not as popular as other greens, it is just as nutritious. One cup of this vegetable provides 106% of vitamin K, 24% for vitamin C and 22% for vitamin A and all for only 4 calories.

Watermelon

Very high water contents.. It tastes great on its own.

Watermelon contains some of almost every nutrient needed and a high amount of vitamin C. There are only 46 calories in one cup watermelon.

. Zucchini

Zucchini is a green type of summer squash. It has a delicate taste that makes it a good addition to recipes.

Spiralizing zucchini into "zoodles" as a substitute for higher carbohydrates noodles is very popular. Zucchini is also low in calories, only 18 per cup.

37. Beverages: Plain water contains no calories. Herbal teas and carbonated waters have zero are a very few calories, while black coffee has just 2 calories per cup.

By choosing these drinks over beverages with sugar, cream or juice can help you reduce your calorie intake even more .

38. Herbs and Spices

Herbs and spices are used to add flavor to foods and are very low in calories. Common herbs : parsley, basil, mint, oregano, cinnamon, paprika, cumin and curry. Most herbs and spices have less than five calories per teaspoon.

There are many foods that are low in calories, but still nutritious.

Most of them are fruits and vegetables that also contain nutrients that benefit your health.

Eating a variety of these foods will provide you with plenty of nutrients for a small amount of calories.

Calories providing the energy that your body needs to function and stay alive.

While there is no evidence to support that negative-calorie foods burn more calories than they provide, foods that are already low in calories may actually provide fewer calories than expected. This is because your body uses energy to digest them.

If you're trying to decrease your total calorie intake, eating more low-calorie foods, such as certain fruits and vegetables, is an easy way to achieve that goal.

Your caloric Intake is important no matter what diet you are on.

List of Superfoods You can use

Eggs

Tomato Sauce

Brussels Sprouts

Prunes

Walnuts

Acai Juice

Apples

Bok Choy

Steel-Cut Oats

Salmon

Avocados

Pumpkin

Spinach

Cauliflower

Scallops

Collard greens

Olives

Brown Rice

Oysters

Edamame

Strawberries

Lentils

Kiwi fruit

whole grains Bran Flakes

Sunflower Seeds

Black Beans

Sardines

Asparagus

Fat-Free Milk

Almond Milk

Coconut Milk

Bananas

Papaya

Brazil Nuts

Seaweed

Tomatoes

Black Raspberries

Garlic

Black Pepper

Fish Oil

Ginger

Peppermint

Pineapple

Sauerkraut

Water

Tart Cherry Juice

Tart Cherries

Spirulina

Parsley best enjoyed by juicing,

wheatgrass best enjoyed by juicing,

Dark Chocolate

Extra-Virgin Olive Oil

Grapefruit

Hemp Seed

Arugula

Blueberries

Extra-Virgin Coconut Oil

Coconut Flour

Carrots

Kale

Dried Mulberries

Cilantro

Buckwheat Pasta

Goji Berries

Pomegranates

Plain yogurt

Onion

Mango

Green Tea

Oranges

Sweet Potato

Turmeric

Figure your ideal daily caloric intake to create the deficit needed to lose weight -

http://www.calculator.net/calorie-calculator.html

Total fat

The dietary reference intake (DRI) for fat in adults is 20% to 35% of total calories from fat. That is about 44 grams to 77 grams of fat per day if you eat 2,000 calories a day. It is recommended to eat more of some types of fats because they provide health benefits. It is recommended to eat less of other types of fat due to the negative impact on health.

Since sources of fat are more calorie-dense, it is important to understand what a serving of a fat is equivalent to. For example, one teaspoon of butter, margarine or mayonnaise is one fat serving. For times when you may not have a measuring spoon available, a visual equivalent of one teaspoon is the tip of your thumb. See below for examples of serving sizes for added fats.

One fat serving is 45 calories, 5 grams of fat:

1 tsp oil, butter, margarine, or mayonnaise

1 Tbsp salad dressing or cream cheese

1 Tbsp reduced-fat mayonnaise or low-fat spread margarine

1.5 to 2 Tbsp reduced fat cream cheese or reduced-fat salad dressing

1 Tbsp seeds (pumpkin, sesame, sunflower)

16 pistachios

10 peanuts

6 almonds, cashews, or mixed nuts

4 pecans or walnut halves

2 Tbsp avocado

1.5 tsp natural peanut butter

8 to 10 olives

Three nutrients — carbohydrate, protein, and fat — contain calories that your body uses for energy. Here's how to balance these nutrients in a healthy diet.

Carbohydrates

Carbohydrate has 4 calories per gram. About 50 to 60 percent of your total daily calories should come from carbohydrate.

Carbohydrate contains the most glucose and gives the quickest form of energy. Your body changes 100 percent of carbohydrate into glucose.

Besides giving your body energy that it uses right away, your body can store carbohydrate in your liver. Your liver stores extra carbohydrate as glycogen and releases it later, when your body needs it. However, there's a limit to the amount of glycogen your liver can store. Once your liver has reached that limit, your body turns the extra carbohydrate into fat.

There are two types of carbohydrate: healthy and not-so-healthy.

Healthy carbohydrates also called complex or slower-acting carbohydrates. Includes multigrain bread, brown rice, lentils, and beans. This type of carbohydrate raises blood sugar slowly and lasts longer. This helps keep you from feeling hungry for a longer time and helps to keep blood sugar levels closer to normal.

Not-so-healthy carbohydrates also known as simple or fast-acting carbohydrates Includes candy, cookies, cake, soda, juice, and sweetened beverages. This type of carbohydrate raises blood sugar levels very quickly, but doesn't last very long. That's why these carbohydrates work well to correct low-blood sugar but don't satisfy hunger as well as healthy carbohydrates.

Proteins

Protein also has 4 calories per gram. In a healthy diet, about 12 to 20 percent of your total daily calories should come from protein.

Your body needs protein for growth, maintenance, and energy. Protein can also be stored and is used mostly by your muscles. Your body changes about 60 percent of protein into glucose.

Protein takes 3 to 4 hours to affect blood sugar levels. When it does have an effect, foods that are mostly protein won't cause much of a rise in blood sugar.

Fats

Fat has the most calories of all the nutrients: 9 calories per gram. In a healthy diet, about 30 percent of total daily calories should come from fat. This means eating about 50 to 80 grams of fat each day. Fat gives the body energy, too, but the body changes only about 10 percent of fat into glucose.

By itself, fat doesn't have much impact on blood sugar. But when you eat fat along with a carbohydrate, it can slow the rise in blood sugar. Since fat also slows down digestion, once your blood sugar does rise, it can keep your blood sugar levels higher for a longer period of time.

There are various types of fat, and some types are better for you than others. Choose mono-unsaturated or poly-unsaturated fat. These fats are liquid at room temperature. Mono-unsaturated fats are especially healthy because they lower the bad cholesterol (LDL) in your blood. These fats include olive, canola, avocado, and nut oils.

Limit saturated and trans-fats. Saturated fats are found in foods that come from animals, such as meat and dairy products. These kinds of fats are solid at room temperature. Hardened fats, such as coconut or palm kernel oils as well as oils that have been hydrogenated, also contain saturated fat. These can damage your heart and arteries.

Trans-fats are found in most processed foods and many fried fast foods, such as French fries. They help food stay fresher longer, but they're just as bad for you as saturated fat.

How Many Fat Grams per Day?

Fat is not the enemy of weight loss. In fact, it's important for good health. It's an essential nutrient that supports healthy skin and hair, facilitates absorption of fat-soluble vitamins, and and supports brain health. However, fat is more calorie-dense than protein or carbohydrates. With 9 calories per gram, you want to eat some – but not too much – when you're trying to lose weight. The type of fat you choose also matters. Unsaturated fats are superior to saturated fats, when it comes to weight loss and your health. The exact number of grams of fat you should eat daily when trying to lose weight depends on your calorie intake goals.

Losing weight requires you to create a calorie deficit. This means you're taking in fewer calories than you burn daily. A daily 500- to 1,000-calorie deficit yields a healthy weight loss of about 1 to 2 pounds per week.

For most women and men, an intake of 1,500 to 2,000 calories represents a lower-calorie diet that supports weight loss. If you need fewer calories to prompt loss, that's OK, but avoid dropping below 1,200 calories as a woman or 1,800 as a man or you risk nutrient deficiencies and a drop in your metabolic rate. Use a weight loss calculator like this one to help kick start healthy weight loss.

Fat Intake When Eating Fewer Calories

You still want a healthy percentage of your daily calorie intake to come from good fats. The Dietary Guidelines for Americans suggest that 25 to 35 percent of your daily calories should come from fat. So, if you consume 1,500 calories on your weight-loss diet, you'll want between 42 and 58 grams of fat daily;, whereas a person eating 2,000 calories would consume between 56 and 78 grams of fat.

To figure the grams according to a specific calorie intake, use the following equation:

(calories per day consumed) x .25 or .35] / 9 = grams of fat to consume per day

Healthy Fats

The types of fats you should emphasize in your diet are those that are unsaturated. Unsaturated fats are found in nuts, seeds, avocados, and fatty fish, such as salmon. Olive oil, flaxseed oil and walnut oil are also good sources.

Unsaturated fats help improve your blood cholesterol, especially when you choose them instead of saturated and Trans fats, explains the American Heart Association. Don't eat them with abandon when you're trying to lose weight, as they're still calorie dense, but make sure the vast majority of your recommended grams of fat come from these healthy fats.

Ideas for including healthy fats in your diet include:

Saute eggs in the morning in olive oil, rather than butter

Add a small amount of avocado to your lunchtime sandwich or salad

Spread almond butter on celery as a snack

Enjoy salmon or mackerel once or twice per week for dinner

Calorie Calculator

http://www.calculator.net/calorie-calculator.htm

Carbohydrates Calculator

https://www.calculator.net/carbohydrate-calculator.html

Fat Calculator

https://www.calculator.net/body-fat-calculator.html

Here are some recipes to get you started

- ## Low carb tomato and basil soup

ingredients

4 portions

800 g Tomato (s), ripe

20 g butter

1 Shallot (n)

1 toe garlic

250 ml of vegetable stock

4 tsp olive oil

8 leaves basil

n. B. sea salt and pepper

Stevia

preparation

Scrap the tomato skin crosswise on a stalk and dip briefly in boiling water, quenching with cold water. Then peel off the tomato skin and then dice the peeled tomatoes.

Peel and finely chop four basil leaves, shallot, and garlic.

Dissolve the butter in a saucepan, add shallots and garlic cubes. After a brief puffing, put the tomato pieces in the pot and steam briefly, then add the broth. Let the soup simmer covered for 10 minutes. Puree the soup and pour it through a fine strainer to remove shallots and tomato pits. Stir in the finely chopped basil. Now season with salt, pepper and possibly sugar or stevia. Spread the soup on four plates, garnish with 1 tsp olive oil and 1 basil leaf.

• Low Carb pizza roll

ingredients

3portions

For the dough:

120 g Quark

3 (S) Egg

120 g Cheese, grated

For covering:

60 g Cheese, grated

n. B. Tomato sauce

n. B. meat

n. B. vegetable

n. B. arugula

preparation

Working time: approx. 10 min. / Cooking time: approx. 30 min. / Level of difficulty: normal / calories p. P .: not specified

Preheat the oven to 170 ° C.

For the ground, mix the quark, eggs and 120 g of cheese in a bowl and season.

Tip the mixture onto the baking sheet with baking paper and smooth it out — Bake for 15 minutes in the oven.

Take out the baking tray and fill the bottom with z. Like tomato sauce, salami, ham, zucchini, mushrooms or corn. Sprinkle with 60 g of cheese and put it back in the oven until the cheese has a nice color.

Allow to cool, sprinkle with rocket and roll gently.

Rolled in aluminum foil, it can be kept in the fridge for several days.

- **Dinner salad**

ingredients

4 portions

1 head   Salad, greener, washed and small plucked

1 Pepper (s), red, cut into strips

3 Tomato (s), wash, cut into eighths

100 g Emmentaler, cut into strips

200 g Pork sausage, cut into strips

3 tbsp walnut oil

4 tbsp cider

1 / 2 tsp sea salt and pepper, to taste

1 bunch   parsley

1 pinch   Stevia

preparation

Working time: approx. 20 min. Rest period: approx. 1 hr. / Difficulty level: simple / calorie p. P .: not specified

Wash and pluck the lettuce, clean the peppers, cut into strips, dice the tomatoes. Cut cheese and sausage into strips, finely chop the parsley and mix everything.

Make the marinade, pour the walnut oil, cider, salt, pepper and sugar over the salad.

Serve with baguette or strong rye bread.

- ## Aepplers sheep cheese - casserole

ingredients

4portions

2 feta cheese

2 Pepper (s), green

4 Tomatoes)

Something basil

Something thyme

pepper

4 (S) Egg

preparation

Working time: approx. 20 min. / Difficulty level: normal / calorie p. P .: not specified

Place the sheep's cheese as a plate in the baking dish. If the slice of feta cheese is too thick, just halve it. Crush the peppers and place over them. Also, give the tomatoes roughly cut. Sprinkle with the spices and finally give the raw eggs (as in fried eggs) over it. Cover with aluminum foil. Bake in the oven at approx. 180 ° C until the eggs are firm if necessary, remove the foil.

- Bad rice salad" from cauliflower

ingredients

4 portions

300 g cauliflower

4 Tomatoes)

1 / 2 Cucumber (n)

1 Spring onions)

200 g Sausage, (poultry meat sausage)

1 Garlic cloves)

3 tbsp yogurt

1 tbsp mayonnaise

2 tbsp Chives, chopped

1 / 2 tsp sea salt

1 pinch pepper

preparation

Working time: approx. 30 min. Rest period: approx. 30 min. / Difficulty level: simple / calorie p. P .: not specified

Grate cauliflower into rice-grain size lightly salts and drain in a sieve over a bowl for at least 30 minutes. Then add cauliflower to a moistened kitchen towel and squeeze out remaining moisture.

Put in a bowl. Cut leftover vegetables and meat sausage into small cubes or rings and add to the cauliflower rasps. Scrape cucumber seeds with a teaspoon first.

From the pressed clove of garlic, yogurt, mayonnaise, chives, and spices to prepare a sauce and mix with the vegetables.

- "Pie" with tuna

ingredients

2

portions

400 g Cream cheese, grainy, light

2 (S) Egg

1 / 2 Pepper (s), red

1 / 2 zucchini

1 big one Onion (n)

1 can Tuna, in its own juice

200 g Cheese, light, grated

sea salt

preparation

Working time: approx. 20 minutes / cooking / baking time: approx. 1 hour / level of difficulty: simple / calories p. P .: not specified

Mix the granular cream cheese with 2 eggs until a smooth mass is obtained. Peel 1 large onion, cut into thin slices or dice and fry in a pan. Clean and dice the pepper and zucchini. Express the tuna well. Mix everything with 50 g - 100 g of grated cheese, add salt and place in a casserole dish. Sprinkle the remaining grated cheese over it.

Approximately Cook for 45-60 minutes at 175 ° C in a preheated oven and brown.

Another variant would be stuffing with steamed mushrooms and 200g cooked ham, also baked with cheese.

- 'The delicacy.'

ingredients

2

portions

2 Chicken breast fillet (s) or turkey breast

salt and pepper

1 ball Mozzarella

Some Basil - leaflets

preparation

Working time: approx. 20 min. / Difficulty level: normal / calorie p. P .: not specified

The chicken breast fillet is first washed and cut into 1-1.5 cm thick slices. Then pepper well on both sides, salt and cover with sliced mozzarella at one end. One big slice is enough for each schnitzel. Make sure that there is still a little space left on edge to prevent the cheese from leaking immediately when frying.

Then 2 - 3 leaves of fresh basil are placed (more or less depending on taste). Now you roll the sandwiches into small rolls and lock them with toothpicks or small skewers. This can be quite tricky, especially with chicken breast fillet and small slices. It is easier with turkey shavings.

The prepared rolls are then only seared and then in a small casserole dish about 10 - 15 minutes (depending on the thickness and oven) at 180 ° C in the oven, so they also durchgaren inside.

If some mozzarella is left over (or you simply like it "cheesier"), you can sprinkle the rolls with diced pieces before baking.

When baking, a little juice comes out, which should be given when serving over the rolls - it tastes delicious. We just eat fresh baguette and green salad. It's a very simple but wonderful recipe.

- ## Good night' cottage cheese

ingredients

1

portions

200 g Cottage cheese, leaner

50 g Tuna (can), natural

20 g linseed

20 ml olive oil

Possibly. Spice (s) of your choice

preparation

Working time: approx. 2 min. / Difficulty level: simple / calorie p. P .: about 465 kcal

Mix all the ingredients in one container and, if you like, season to taste. I put the bowl in the fridge before eating, so that the mass is a little firmer.

The snack is extremely filling due to the protein/fat combination. The cottage cheese is suitable for athletes especially as a snack before going to sleep because the contained casein (whey protein) is processed quite slowly and thus provides the body throughout the night on protein to build muscle. The fat also supports this effect.

The snack provides approximately:

465 kcal

4 g carbohydrates

27 g fat (excluding monounsaturated and polyunsaturated)

38 g protein

By omitting the olive oil, one can save something here.

The snack may sound a bit strange, but I always enjoy new food every night! Just try it.

- ## 15 minutes - Schaschli pot

ingredients

4

 portions

500 g   Pork, in cubes

250 g   Bacon, (or bacon)

3 Pepper (s), colorful

2 Onion (n)

1 zucchini

250 g mushrooms

2 bottles Sauce (gypsy sauce)

100 ml   tomato ketchup

175 ml of wate

rsea salt and pepper

curry powder

preparation

Working time: approx. 20 min. / Difficulty level: simple / calorie p. P .: not specified

Cut all ingredients into big pieces. Fry the onions and bacon neatly in a large roasting pan. Put the onions and bacon on the lid and fry the meat on all sides. Add vegetables and onion/bacon. Add 175 ml of water, gypsy sauce, ketchup and spices and in the closed roaster for 1.5 hours at 200 ° on the bottom rail in the oven.

With pasta, rice, or baguette.

- **3 small protein pancakes, low carb**

ingredients

1

 portions

70 g oatmeal

2 protein

10 g Protein powder (whey)

Almond milk (almond drink) or soy milk

Cinnamon powder to taste

Stevia to taste

1 / 2 tsp Lemon peel

preparation

Working time: approx. 15 min. / Cooking time: approx. 10 min. / Level of difficulty: simple / calorie p. P .: not specified

Grind oatmeal to flour. Beat egg whites until stiff. Mix all ingredients, except the egg whites, to a dough, adding the almond milk while stirring until the desired consistency is achieved. Then carefully fold in the egg whites. Bake the dough in a pan.

Tip: with quark and forest fruits, the pancakes taste particularly delicious. I mixed the quark with some almond milk and the juice of frozen berries and made the berries on the pancakes.

Have a happy weight loss.

If you Get A Chance go and leave a book review. It only takes a few minutes and I promise it's not painful.

My site.

https://glensdieting.com/wpx2